Mediterranean Diet Cookbook

50 Delicious and Easy Recipes for a Lifelong Health

By Terri Armstrong

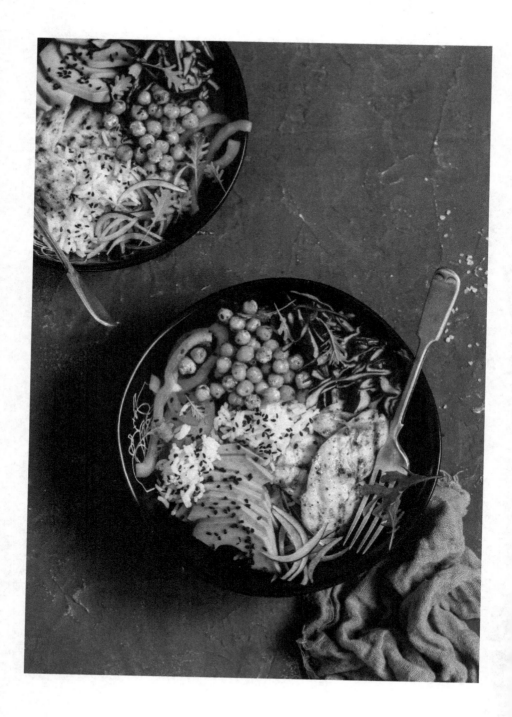

Table of Contents

4

Introduction

Mediterranean diet is based on the eating habits of the inhabitants of the regions along the Mediterranean Sea, mostly from Italy, Spain and Greece; it is considered more a life style then a diet, in fact it also promotes physical activity and proper liquid (mostly water) consumption.

Depending on fresh seasonal local foods there are no strict rules, because of the many cultural differences, but there are some common factors.

Mediterranean diet has become famous for its ability to reduce heart disease and obesity, thanks to the low consumption of unhealthy fats that increase blood glucose.

Mediterranean diet is mostly plant based, so it's rich of antioxidants; vegetables, fruits like apple and grapes, olive oil, whole grains, herbs, beans and nuts are consumed in large quantities.

Moderate amounts of poultry, eggs, dairy and seafood are also common aliments, accompanied by a little bit of red wine (some studies say that in small amount it helps to stay healthy).

Red meat and sweets like cookies and cakes are accepted but are more limited in quantity.

Foods to avoid:

- refined grains, such as white bread and pasta
- dough containing white flour refined oils (even canola oil and soybean oil)
- foods with added sugars (like pastries, sodas, and candies)

processed meats processed or packaged foods

Chapter 1: Breakfast and Snack Recipes

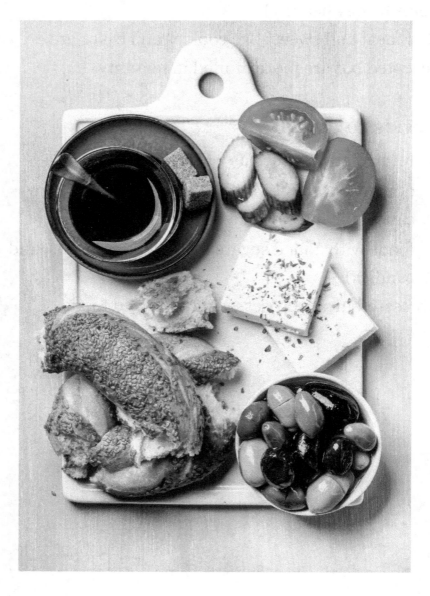

Herbed Goat Cheese Dip

Servings: 4 | Cooking: 0 min

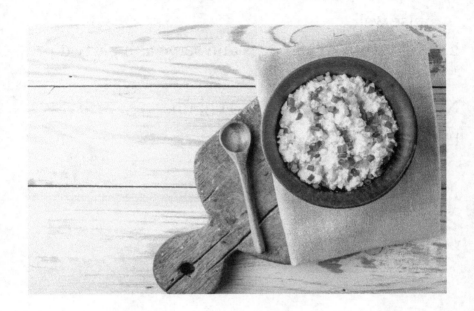

Ingredients

- ¼ cup mixed parsley, chopped
- ¼ cup chives, chopped
- 8 ounces goat cheese, soft
- Salt and black pepper to the taste
- A drizzle of olive oil

Directions

1. In your food processor mix the goat cheese with the parsley and the rest of the ingredients and pulse well.
2. Divide into small bowls and serve as a party dip.

Nutrition: calories 245; fat 11.3; fiber 4.5; carbs 8.9; protein 11.2

Italian Wheatberry Cakes

Servings: 6 | Cooking: 15 min

Ingredients

- 1 cup wheatberry, cooked
- 2 eggs
- ¼ cup ground chicken
- 1 tablespoon wheat flour, whole grain
- 1 teaspoon Italian seasoning
- 1 tablespoon olive oil
- 1 teaspoon salt

Directions

1. In the mixing bowl mix up together wheatberry and ground chicken.
2. Crack eggs in the mixture.
3. Then add wheat flour, Italian seasoning, and salt.
4. Mix up the mass with the help of the spoon until homogenous.
5. Then make burgers and freeze them in the freezer for 20 minutes.
6. Heat up olive oil in the skillet.

7. Place frozen burgers in the hot oil and roast them for 4 minutes from each side over the high heat.
8. Then cook burgers for 10 minutes more over the medium heat. Flip them onto another side from time to time.

Nutrition: calories 97; fat 5.7; fiber 1.5; carbs 9.2; protein 5.2

Healthy Kidney Bean Dip

Servings: 6 | Cooking: 10 min

Ingredients

- 1 cup dry white kidney beans, soaked overnight and drained
- 1 tbsp fresh lemon juice
- 2 tbsp water
- 1/2 cup coconut yogurt
- 1 roasted garlic clove
- 1 tbsp olive oil
- 1/4 tsp cayenne
- 1 tsp dried parsley
- Pepper
- Salt

Directions

1. Add soaked beans and 1 3/4 cups of water into the instant pot.
2. Seal pot with lid and cook on high for 10 minutes.
3. Once done, allow to release pressure naturally. Remove lid.

4. Drain beans well and transfer them into the food processor.
5. Add remaining ingredients into the food processor and process until smooth.
6. Serve and enjoy.

Nutrition: Calories 136 Fat 3.2 g Carbohydrates 20 g Sugar 2.1 g Protein 7.7 g Cholesterol 0 mg

Lentils Spread

Servings: 12 | Cooking: 0 min

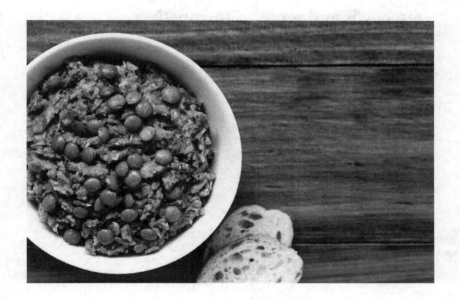

Ingredients

- 1 garlic clove, minced
- 12 ounces canned lentils, drained and rinsed
- 1 teaspoon oregano, dried
- ¼ teaspoon basil, dried
- 3 tablespoons olive oil
- 1 tablespoon balsamic vinegar
- Salt and black pepper to the taste

Directions

1. In a blender, combine the lentils with the garlic
   and the rest of the ingredients, pulse well, divide
   into bowls and serve as an appetizer.

Nutrition: calories 287; fat 9.5; fiber 3.5; carbs 15.3;
protein 9.3

Chickpeas Spread

Servings: 7 | Cooking: 45 min

Ingredients

- 1 cup chickpeas, soaked
- 6 cups of water
- ½ cup lemon juice
- 3 tablespoon olive oil
- 1 teaspoon salt
- 1/3 teaspoon harissa

Directions

1. Combine together chickpeas and water and boil for 45 minutes or until chickpeas are tender.
2. Then transfer chickpeas in the food processor.
3. Add 1 cup of chickpeas water and lemon juice.
4. After this, add salt and harissa.
5. Blend the hummus until it is smooth and fluffy.
6. Add olive oil and pulse it for 10 seconds more.
7. Transfer the cooked hummus in the bowl and store it in the fridge up to 2 days.

Nutrition: calories 160; fat 7.9; fiber 5. carbs 17.8; protein 5.7

Lime Yogurt Dip

Servings: 4 | Cooking: 0 min

Ingredients

- 1 large cucumber, trimmed
- 3 oz Greek yogurt
- 1 teaspoon olive oil
- 3 tablespoons fresh dill, chopped
- 1 tablespoon lime juice
- ¾ teaspoon salt
- 1 garlic clove, minced

Directions

1. Grate the cucumber and squeeze the juice from it.
2. Then place the squeezed cucumber in the bowl.
3. Add Greek yogurt, olive oil, dill, lime juice, salt, and minced garlic.
4. Mix up the mixture until homogenous.
5. Store tzaziki in the fridge up to 2 days.

Nutrition: calories 44; fat 1.8; fiber 0.7; carbs 5.1; protein 3.2

Almond Bowls

Servings: 5 | Cooking: 15 min

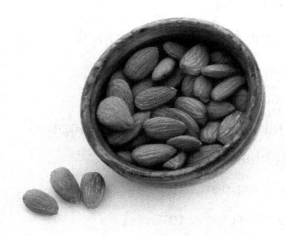

Ingredients

- 1 cup almonds
- 3 tablespoons salt
- 2 cups of water

Directions

1. Bring water to boil.
2. After this, add 2 tablespoons of salt in water and stir it.

3. When salt is dissolved, add almonds and let them soak for at least 1 hour.
4. Meanwhile, line the tray with baking paper and preheat oven to 350F.
5. Dry the soaked almonds with a paper towel well and arrange them in one layer in the tray.
6. Sprinkle buts with remaining salt.
7. Bake the snack for 15 minutes. Mix it from time to time with the help of the spatula or spoon.

Nutrition: calories 110; fat 9.5; fiber 2.4; carbs 4.1; protein 4

Beet Spread

Servings: 4 | Cooking: 35 min

Ingredients

- 1 tablespoon pumpkin puree
- 1 beet, peeled
- 1 teaspoon tahini paste
- ½ teaspoon sesame seeds
- 1 teaspoon paprika
- 1 tablespoon olive oil
- ¼ cup water, boiled
- 1 tablespoon lime juice
- ½ teaspoon salt

Directions

1. Place beet in the oven and bake it at 375F for 35 minutes.
2. Then chop it roughly and put in the food processor.
3. Blend the beet until smooth.
4. After this, add tahini paste, pumpkin puree, paprika, olive oil, water, lime juice, and salt.

5. Blend the hummus until smooth and fluffy.
6. Then transfer the appetizer in the bowl and sprinkle with sesame seeds.

Nutrition: calories 99; fat 8.6; fiber 1.6; carbs 3.9; protein 2.1

Calamari Mediterranean

Servings: 2 | Cooking: 10 min

Ingredients

- 1 tablespoon Italian parsley
- 1 teaspoon ancho chili, chopped
- 1 teaspoon cumin
- 1 teaspoon red pepper flakes
- 1/2 cup white wine
- 2 cups calamari
- 2 medium plum tomatoes, diced
- 2 tablespoons capers
- 2 tablespoons garlic cloves, roasted
- 2 tablespoons olive oil
- 2 tablespoons unsalted butter
- 3 tablespoons lime juice
- Salt

Directions

1. Heat a sauté pan. Add the oil, garlic, and the calamari; sauté for 1 minute. Add the capers, red

pepper flakes, cumin, ancho chili and the diced tomatoes; cook for 1 minute.

2. Add the wine and the lime juice; simmer for 4 minutes.
3. Stir in the butter, parsley, and the salt; continue cooking until the sauce is thick.
4. Serve with whole-wheat French bread.

Nutrition:308.8 cal., 25.7 g total fat (9.3 sat. fat), 30.5 mg chol., 267.8 mg sodium, 10.2 g total carbs., 1.7 g fiber, 2.8 g sugar, and 1.9 g protein.

Cheddar Dip

Servings: 6 | Cooking: 10 min

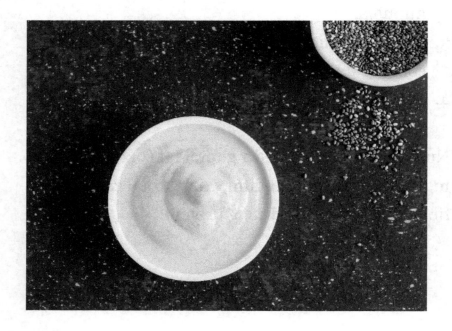

Ingredients

- 1 cup Cheddar cheese
- ¼ cup cilantro, chopped
- 1 chili pepper, chopped
- 1 teaspoon garlic powder
- ¼ cup milk

Directions

1. Bring the milk to boil.
2. Then add Cheddar cheese in the milk and simmer the mixture for 2 minutes. Stir it constantly.
3. After this, add cilantro, chili pepper, and garlic powder. Mix up the mixture well. If it doesn't get a smooth texture, use the hand blender to blend the mass.
4. It is recommended to serve the dip when it gets the room temperature.

Nutrition: calories 83; fat 6.5; fiber 0.1; carbs 1.2; protein 5.1

Chapter 2: Lunch & Dinner Recipes

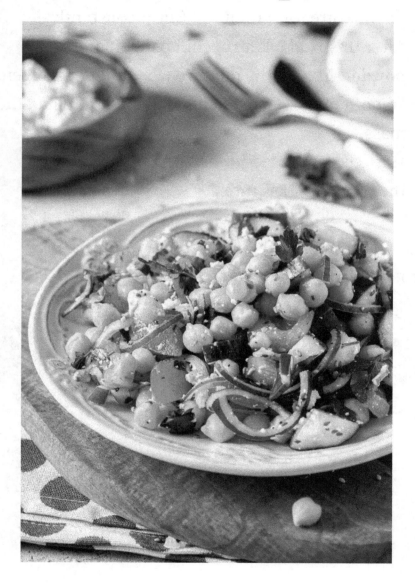

Beef Stuffed Bell Peppers

Servings: 6 | Cooking: 1 Hour

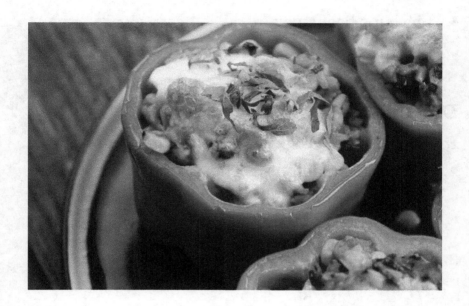

Ingredients

- 6 red bell peppers
- 1 pound ground beef
- 2 sweet onions, chopped
- 1 garlic cloves, minced
- 1 carrot, grated
- 1 celery stalk, finely chopped
- 1 tablespoon pesto sauce
- 2 tablespoons tomato paste

- ½ cup white rice
- Salt and pepper to taste
- 1 cup tomato juice
- 1 ½ cups beef stock
- 1 thyme sprig

Directions

1. Place the thyme sprig at the bottom of a pot.
2. Mix the beef, onions, garlic, carrot, celery, pesto sauce and tomato paste, as well as rice, salt and pepper in a bowl.
3. Cut the top of each bell pepper and remove the vines.
4. Stuff the bell peppers with the beef mixture and place them in the pot.
5. Pour in the tomato juice and stock and cover with a lid.
6. Cook on low heat for 45 minutes.
7. Serve the bell peppers warm and fresh.

Nutrition: Calories:280 Fat:6.5g Protein:27.2g Carbohydrates:27.1g

Stuffed Eggplants

Servings: 4 | Cooking: 35 min

Ingredients

- 2 eggplants, halved lengthwise and 2/3 of the flesh scooped out
- 3 tablespoons olive oil
- 1 red onion, chopped
- 2 garlic cloves, minced
- 1 pint white mushrooms, sliced
- 2 cups kale, torn
- 2 cups quinoa, cooked
- 1 tablespoon thyme, chopped
- Zest and juice of 1 lemon
- Salt and black pepper to the taste
- ½ cup Greek yogurt
- 3 tablespoons parsley, chopped

Directions

1. Rub the inside of each eggplant half with half of the oil and arrange them on a baking sheet lined with parchment paper.

2. Heat up a pan with the rest of the oil over medium heat, add the onion and the garlic and sauté for 5 minutes.
3. Add the mushrooms and cook for 5 minutes more.
4. Add the kale, salt, pepper, thyme, lemon zest and juice, stir, cook for 5 minutes more and take off the heat.
5. Stuff the eggplant halves with the mushroom mix, introduce them in the oven and bake 400 degrees F for 20 minutes.
6. Divide the eggplants between plates, sprinkle the parsley and the yogurt on top and serve for lunch.

Nutrition: calories 512; fat 16.4; fiber 17.5; carbs 78; protein 17.2

Mushroom Pilaf

Servings: 4 | Cooking: 50 min

Ingredients

- 2 tablespoons olive oil
- 1 shallot, chopped
- 2 garlic cloves, minced
- 1 pound button mushrooms
- 1 cup brown rice
- 2 cups chicken stock
- 1 bay leaf
- 1 thyme sprig
- Salt and pepper to taste

Directions

1. Heat the oil in a skillet and stir in the shallot and garlic. Cook for 2 minutes until softened and fragrant.
2. Add the mushrooms and rice and cook for 5 minutes.

3. Add the stock, bay leaf and thyme, as well as salt and pepper and continue cooking for 20 more minutes on low heat.
4. Serve the pilaf warm and fresh.

Nutrition: Calories:265 Fat:8.9g Protein:7.6g Carbohydrates:41.2g

Cream Cheese Artichoke Mix

Servings: 6 | Cooking: 45 min

Ingredients

- 4 sheets matzo
- ½ cup artichoke hearts, canned
- 1 cup cream cheese
- 1 cup spinach, chopped
- ½ teaspoon salt
- 1 teaspoon ground black pepper
- 3 tablespoons fresh dill, chopped
- 3 eggs, beaten
- 1 teaspoon canola oil
- ½ cup cottage cheese

Directions

1. In the bowl combine together cream cheese, spinach, salt, ground black pepper, dill, and cottage cheese.
2. Pour canola oil in the skillet, add artichoke hearts and roast them for 2-3 minutes over the medium heat. Stir them from time to time.

3. Then add roasted artichoke hearts in the cheese mixture.
4. Add eggs and stir until homogenous.
5. Place one sheet of matzo in the casserole mold.
6. Then spread it with cheese mixture generously.
7. Cover the cheese layer with the second sheet of matzo.
8. Repeat the steps till you use all ingredients.
9. Then preheat oven to 360F.
10. Bake matzo mina for 40 minutes.
11. Cut the cooked meal into the servings.

Nutrition: calories 272; fat 17.3; fiber 4.3; carbs 20.2; protein 11.8

Caramelized Shallot Steaks

Servings: 6 | Cooking: 45 min

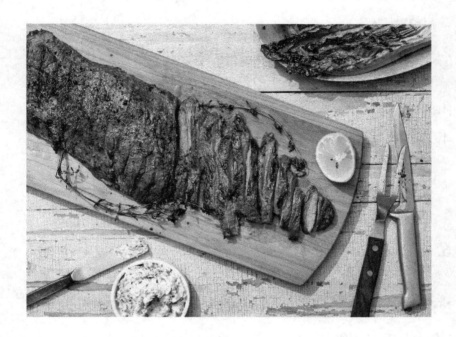

Ingredients

- 6 flank steaks
- Salt and pepper to taste
- 1 teaspoon dried oregano
- 1 teaspoon dried basil
- 6 shallots, sliced
- 4 tablespoons olive oil
- ¼ cup dry white wine

Directions

1. Season the steaks with salt, pepper, oregano and basil.
2. Heat a grill pan over medium flame and place the steaks on the grill.
3. Cook on each side for 6-7 minutes.
4. Heat the oil in a skillet and stir in the shallots. Cook for 15 minutes, stirring often, until the shallots are caramelized.
5. Add the wine and cook for another 5 minutes.
6. Serve the steaks with shallots.

Nutrition: Calories:258 Fat:16.3g Protein:23.5g Carbohydrates:2.1g

Chapter 3: Meat Recipes

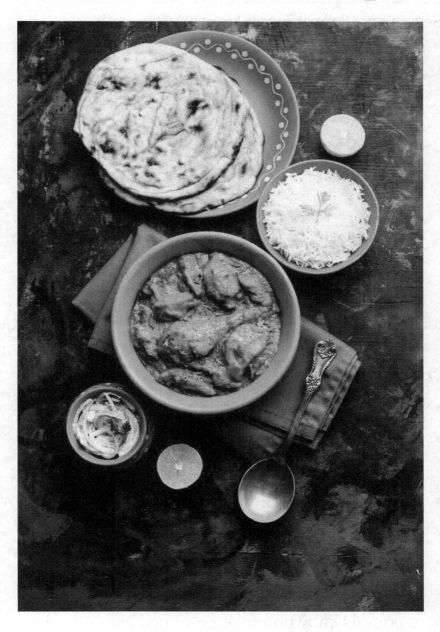

Lemony Lamb And Potatoes

Servings: 4 | Cooking: 2 Hours And 10 min

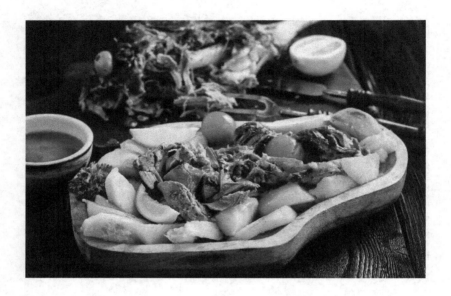

Ingredients

- 2 pound lamb meat, cubed
- 2 tablespoons olive oil
- 2 springs rosemary, chopped
- 2 tablespoons parsley, chopped
- 1 tablespoon lemon rind, grated
- 3 garlic cloves, minced
- 2 tablespoons lemon juice
- 2 pounds baby potatoes, scrubbed and halved

- 1 cup veggie stock

Directions

1. In a roasting pan, combine the meat with the oil and the rest of the ingredients, introduce in the oven and bake at 400 degrees F for 2 hours and 10 minutes.
2. Divide the mix between plates and serve.

Nutrition: calories 302; fat 15.2; fiber 10.6; carbs 23.3; protein 15.2

Cumin Lamb Mix

Servings: 2 | Cooking: 10 min

Ingredients

- 2 lamb chops (3.5 oz each)
- 1 tablespoon olive oil
- 1 teaspoon ground cumin
- ½ teaspoon salt

Directions

1. Rub the lamb chops with ground cumin and salt.
2. Then sprinkle them with olive oil.
3. Let the meat marinate for 10 minutes.
4. After this, preheat the skillet well.
5. Place the lamb chops in the skillet and roast them for 10 minutes. Flip the meat on another side from time to time to avoid burning.

Nutrition: calories 384; fat 33.2; fiber 0.1; carbs 0.5; protein 19.2

Almond Lamb Chops

Servings: 4 | Cooking: 20 min

Ingredients

- 1 teaspoon almond butter
- 2 teaspoons minced garlic
- 1 teaspoon butter, softened
- ½ teaspoon salt
- ½ teaspoon chili flakes
- ½ teaspoon ground paprika
- 12 oz lamb chop

Directions

1. Churn together minced garlic, butter, salt, chili flakes, and ground paprika.
2. Carefully rub every lamb chop with the garlic mixture.
3. Toss almond butter in the skillet and melt it.
4. Place the lamb chops in the melted almond butter and roast them for 20 minutes (for 10 minutes from each side) over the medium-low heat.

Nutrition: calories 194; fat 9.5; fiber 0.5; carbs 1.4; protein 24.9

Pork And Figs Mix

Servings: 4 | Cooking: 40 min

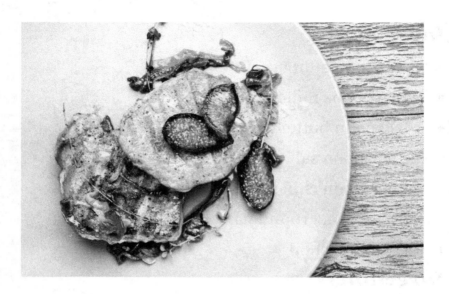

Ingredients

- 3 tablespoons avocado oil
- 1 and ½ pounds pork stew meat, roughly cubed
- Salt and black pepper to the taste
- 1 cup red onions, chopped
- 1 cup figs, dried and chopped
- 1 tablespoon ginger, grated
- 1 tablespoon garlic, minced
- 1 cup canned tomatoes, crushed

- 2 tablespoons parsley, chopped

Directions

1. Heat up a pot with the oil over medium-high heat, add the meat and brown for 5 minutes.
2. Add the onions and sauté for 5 minutes more.
3. Add the rest of the ingredients, bring to a simmer and cook over medium heat for 30 minutes more.
4. Divide the mix between plates and serve.

Nutrition: calories 309; fat 16; fiber 10.4; carbs 21.1; protein 34.2

Lamb Chops

Servings: 1 Chop | Cooking: 6 min

Ingredients

- 6 (3/4-in.-thick) lamb chops
- 2 TB. fresh rosemary, finely chopped
- 3 TB. minced garlic
- 1 tsp. salt
- 1 tsp. ground black pepper
- 3 TB. extra-virgin olive oil

Directions

1. In a large bowl, combine lamb chops, rosemary, garlic, salt, black pepper, and extra-virgin olive oil until chops are evenly coated. Let chops marinate at room temperature for at least 25 minutes.
2. Preheat a grill to medium heat.
3. Place chops on the grill, and cook for 3 minutes per side for medium well.
4. Serve warm.

Chapter 4: Poultry Recipes

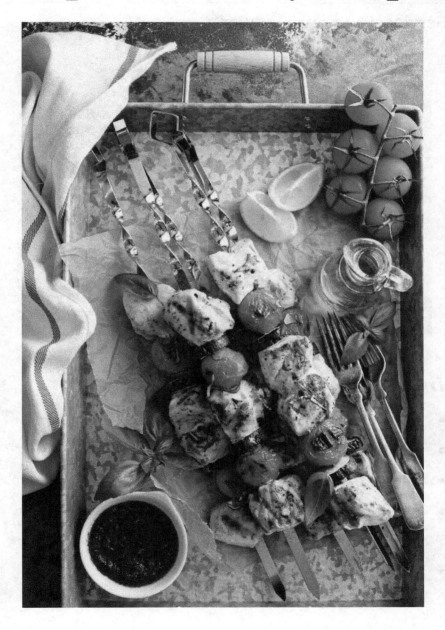

Chicken And Tomato Pan

Servings: 4 | Cooking: 30 min

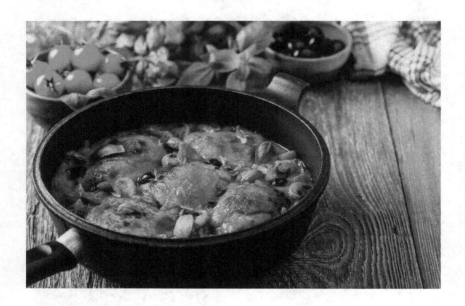

Ingredients

- 12 oz chicken fillet
- 4 kalamata olives, chopped
- 4 tomatoes, chopped
- 1 yellow onion, diced
- 1 tablespoon olive oil
- ½ cup of water

Directions

1. Pour olive oil in the saucepan.
2. Add diced yellow onion and cook it for 5 minutes. Stir it from time to time.
3. After this, add olives and chopped tomatoes. Mix up well and cook vegetables for 5 minutes more.
4. Meanwhile, chop the chicken fillet.
5. Add the chicken fillet in the tomato mixture and mix up.
6. Close the lid.
7. Simmer the chicken for 20 minutes over the medium heat.

Nutrition: calories 230; fat 10.6; fiber 2.2; carbs 7.6; protein 26

Smoked And Hot Turkey Mix

Servings: 4 | Cooking: 40 min

Ingredients

- 1 red onion, sliced
- 1 big turkey breast, skinless, boneless and roughly cubed
- 1 tablespoon smoked paprika
- 2 chili peppers, chopped
- Salt and black pepper to the taste
- 2 tablespoons olive oil
- ½ cup chicken stock
- 1 tablespoon parsley, chopped
- 1 tablespoon cilantro, chopped

Directions

1. Grease a roasting pan with the oil, add the turkey, onion, paprika and the rest of the ingredients, toss, introduce in the oven and bake at 425 degrees F for 40 minutes.
2. Divide the mix between plates and serve right away.

Nutrition: calories 310; fat 18.4; fiber 10.4; carbs 22.3; protein 33.4

Chicken With Artichokes

Servings: 3 | Cooking: 30 min

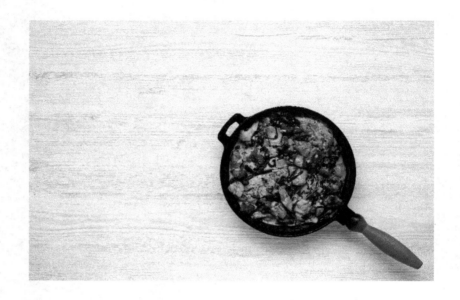

Ingredients

- 1 can artichoke hearts, chopped
- 12 oz chicken fillets (3 oz each fillet)
- 1 teaspoon avocado oil
- ½ teaspoon ground thyme
- ½ teaspoon white pepper
- 1/3 cup water
- 1/3 cup shallot, roughly chopped
- 1 lemon, sliced

Directions

1. Mix up together chicken fillets, artichoke hearts, avocado oil, ground thyme, white pepper, and shallot.
2. Line the baking tray with baking paper and place the chicken fillet mixture in it.
3. Then add sliced lemon and water.
4. Bake the meal for 30 minutes at 375F. Stir the ingredients during cooking to avoid burning.

Nutrition: calories 263; fat 8.8; fiber 3.7; carbs 10.9; protein 35.3

Brown Rice, Chicken And Scallions

Servings: 4 | Cooking: 30 min

Ingredients

- 1 and ½ cups brown rice
- 3 cups chicken stock
- 2 tablespoon balsamic vinegar
- 1 pound chicken breast, boneless, skinless and cubed
- 6 scallions, chopped
- Salt and black pepper to the taste
- 1 tablespoon sweet paprika
- 2 tablespoons avocado oil

Directions

1. Heat up a pan with the oil over medium-high heat, add the chicken and brown for 5 minutes.
2. Add the scallions and sauté for 5 minutes more.
3. Add the rice and the rest of the ingredients, bring to a simmer and cook over medium heat for 20 minutes.
4. Stir the mix, divide everything between plates and serve.

Nutrition: calories 300; fat 9.2; fiber 11.8; carbs 18.6; protein 23.8

Greek Chicken Bites

Servings: 6 | Cooking: 20 min

Ingredients

- 1-pound chicken fillet
- 1 tablespoon Greek seasoning
- 1 teaspoon sesame oil
- ½ teaspoon salt
- 1 teaspoon balsamic vinegar

Directions

1. Cut the chicken fingers on small tenders (fingers) and sprinkle them with Greek seasoning, salt, and balsamic vinegar. Mix up well with the help of the fingertips.
2. Then sprinkle chicken with sesame oil and shake gently.
3. Line the baking tray with parchment.
4. Place the marinated chicken fingers in the tray in one layer.
5. Bake the chicken fingers for 20 minutes at 355F. Flip them on another side after 10 minutes of cooking.

Nutrition: calories 154; fat 6.4; fiber 0; carbs 0.8; protein 22

Chapter 5: Fish and Seafood Recipes

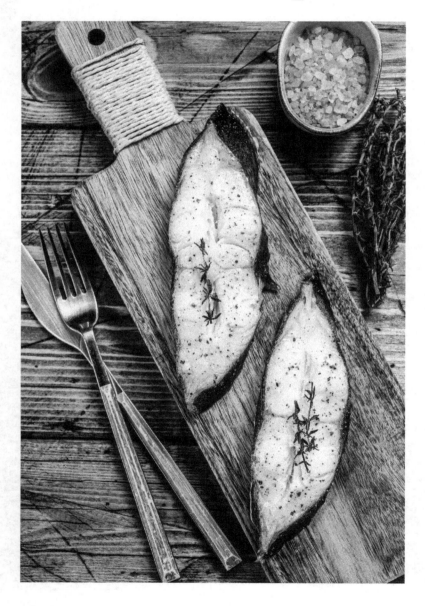

Creamy Scallops

Servings: 4 | Cooking: 7 min

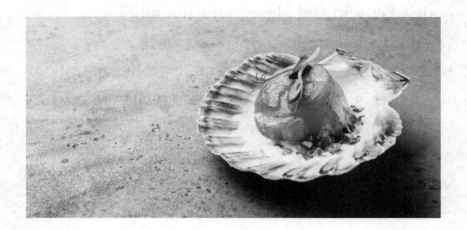

Ingredients

- ½ cup heavy cream
- 1 teaspoon fresh rosemary
- ½ teaspoon dried cumin
- ½ teaspoon garlic, diced
- 8 oz bay scallops
- 1 teaspoon olive oil
- ½ teaspoon salt
- ¼ teaspoon chili flakes

Directions

1. Preheat olive oil in the skillet until hot.
2. Then sprinkle scallops with salt, chili flakes, and dried cumin and place in the hot oil.
3. Add fresh rosemary and diced garlic.
4. Roast the scallops for 2 minutes from each side.
5. After this, add heavy cream and bring the mixture to boil. Boil it for 1 minute.

Nutrition: calories 114; fat 7.3; fiber 0.2; carbs 2.2; protein 9.9

Fish And Rice (sayadieh)

Servings: 1 Cup | Cooking: 1½hours

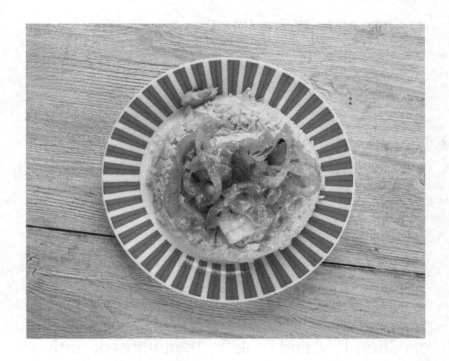

Ingredients

- 1 lb. whitefish fillets (cod, tilapia, or haddock)
- 2 tsp. salt
- 2 tsp. ground black pepper
- 1/4 cup plus 2 TB. extra-virgin olive oil
- 2 large yellow onions, sliced
- 5 cups water

- 1 tsp. turmeric
- 1 tsp. ground coriander
- 1/2 tsp. ground cumin
- 1/4 tsp. ground cinnamon
- 2 cups basmati rice
- 1/2 cup sliced almonds

Directions

1. Season both sides of whitefish with 1 teaspoon salt and 1 teaspoon black pepper.
2. In a skillet over medium heat, heat 1/4 cup extra-virgin olive oil. Add fish, and cook for 3 minutes per side. Remove fish from the pan.
3. Add yellow onions to the skillet, reduce heat to medium-low, and cook for 15 minutes or until golden brown and caramelized.
4. In a 3-quart pot over medium heat, add 1/2 of cooked onions, water, turmeric, coriander, cumin, cinnamon, remaining 1 teaspoon salt, and remaining 1 teaspoon black pepper. Simmer for 20 minutes.
5. Add basmati rice, cover, and cook for 30 minutes.

6. Cut fish into 1/2-inch pieces, fluff rice, and gently fold fish into rice. Cover and cook for 10 more minutes.

7. Remove from heat, and let sit for 10 minutes before serving.

8. Meanwhile, in a small saucepan over low heat, heat remaining 2 tablespoons extra-virgin olive oil. Add almonds, and toast for 3 minutes.

9. Spoon fish and rice onto a serving plate, top with remaining onions and toasted almonds, and serve.

Creamy Bacon-fish Chowder

Servings: 8 | Cooking: 30 min

Ingredients

- 1 1/2 lbs. cod
- 1 1/2 tsp dried thyme
- 1 large onion, chopped
- 1 medium carrot, coarsely chopped
- 1 tbsp butter, cut into small pieces
- 1 tsp salt, divided
- 3 1/2 cups baking potato, peeled and cubed
- 3 slices uncooked bacon
- 3/4 tsp freshly ground black pepper, divided
- 4 1/2 cups water
- 4 bay leaves
- 4 cups 2% reduced-fat milk

Directions

1. In a large skillet, add the water and bay leaves and let it simmer. Add the fish. Cover and let it simmer some more until the flesh flakes easily with fork. Remove the fish from the skillet and cut into large pieces. Set aside the cooking liquid.

2. Place Dutch oven in medium heat and cook the bacon until crisp. Remove the bacon and reserve the bacon drippings. Crush the bacon and set aside.
3. Stir potato, onion and carrot in the pan with the bacon drippings, cook over medium heat for 10 minutes. Add the cooking liquid, bay leaves, 1/2 tsp salt, 1/4 tsp pepper and thyme, let it boil. Lower the heat and let simmer for 10 minutes. Add the milk and butter, simmer until the potatoes becomes tender, but do not boil. Add the fish, 1/2 tsp salt, 1/2 tsp pepper. Remove the bay leaves.
4. Serve sprinkled with the crushed bacon.

Nutrition: Calories per serving: 400; Carbs: 34.5g; Protein: 20.8g; Fat: 19.7g

Healthy Poached Trout

Servings: 2 | Cooking: 10 min

Ingredients

- 1 8-oz boneless, skin on trout fillet
- 2 cups chicken broth or water
- 2 leeks, halved
- 6-8 slices lemon
- salt and pepper to taste

Directions

1. On medium fire, place a large nonstick skillet and arrange leeks and lemons on pan in a layer. Cover with soup stock or water and bring to a simmer.
2. Meanwhile, season trout on both sides with pepper and salt. Place trout on simmering pan of water. Cover and cook until trout is flaky, around 8 minutes.
3. In a serving platter, spoon leek and lemons on bottom of plate, top with trout and spoon sauce into plate. Serve and enjoy.

Nutrition: Calories per serving: 360.2; Protein: 13.8g; Fat: 7.5g; Carbs: 51.5g

Creamy Curry Salmon

Servings: 2 | Cooking: 20 min

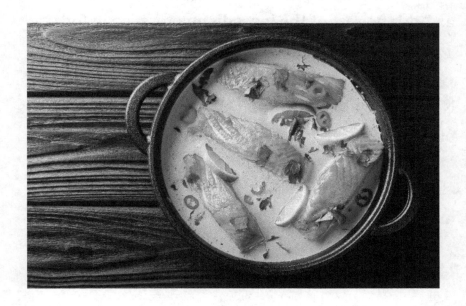

Ingredients

- 2 salmon fillets, boneless and cubed
- 1 tablespoon olive oil
- 1 tablespoon basil, chopped
- Sea salt and black pepper to the taste
- 1 cup Greek yogurt
- 2 teaspoons curry powder
- 1 garlic clove, minced
- ½ teaspoon mint, chopped

Directions

1. Heat up a pan with the oil over medium-high heat, add the salmon and cook for 3 minutes.
2. Add the rest of the ingredients, toss, cook for 15 minutes more, divide between plates and serve.

Nutrition: calories 284; fat 14.1; fiber 8.5; carbs 26.7; protein 31.4

Chapter 6: Salads & Side Dishes

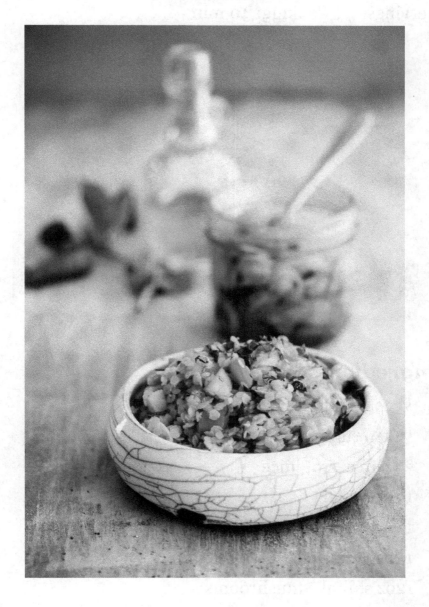

Kasha With Onions And Mushrooms

Servings: 4 | Cooking: 40 min

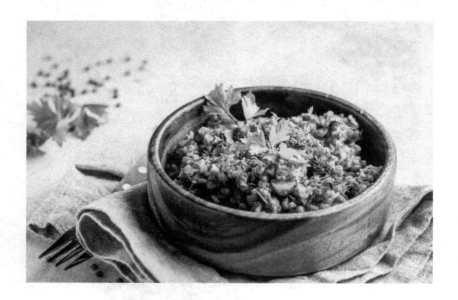

Ingredients

- ½ tsp pepper
- ½ tsp rubbed sage
- ¾ cup carrot juice
- 1 cup water
- 1 cup whole grain kasha
- 1 tbsp olive oil
- 12oz shiitake mushrooms

- 2 large onions, thinly sliced
- 2 tsp sugar
- Salt to taste

Directions

1. In a large skillet, heat oil over medium high heat and add onions and sugar. Cook until the onions are brown.
2. Add the sage, mushrooms and pepper stir constantly until the mushrooms are tender. Set aside.
3. In the same skillet, place kasha and cook over medium heat. Stir constantly until lightly toasted.
4. Combine carrot juice, water and salt in a saucepan and bring to a boil over medium heat.
5. Add kasha and cook until tender.
6. Fluff with fork and transfer the contents to the skillet with the onion and sugar mixture.
7. Toss until well combined.
8. Serve and enjoy.

Nutrition: Calories: 254.5; Carbs: 46.8 g; Protein: 6.7g; Fat: 4.5g

Chickpea Alfredo Sauce

Servings: 4 | Cooking: 0 min

Ingredients

- ¼ teaspoon ground nutmeg
- ¼ teaspoon sea salt or to taste
- 1 clove garlic minced
- 2 cups chickpeas, rinsed and drained
- 1 tablespoon white miso paste
- 1-½ cups water
- 2 tablespoons lemon juice
- 3 tablespoons Nutritional yeast

Directions

1. Add all ingredients in a blender.
2. Puree until smooth and creamy.

Nutrition: Calories per serving: 123; Protein: 6.2g; Carbs: 20.2g; Fat: 2.4g

Lime-cilantro Rice Chipotle Style

Servings: 10 | Cooking: 17 min

Ingredients

- 1 can vegetable broth
- ¾ cup water
- 2 tablespoons canola oil
- 3 tablespoons juice of lime juice
- 2 cups long grain white rice, rinsed
- Zest of 1 lime
- ½ cup cilantro, chopped
- ½ teaspoon salt

Directions

1. Place everything in the pot and give a good stir.
2. Give a good stir and close the lid.
3. Seal off the vent.
4. Press the Rice button and adjust the cooking time to 17 minutes.
5. Do natural pressure release.
6. Fluff the rice before serving.
7. Once cooled, evenly divide into serving size, keep in your preferred container, and refrigerate until ready to eat.

<u>Nutrition: Calories per serving: 166; Carbohydrates: 31.2g; Protein:2.7 g; Fat: 3.1g</u>

Lentils And Rice (mujaddara With Rice)

Servings: 1 Cup | Cooking: 1 Hour 10 min

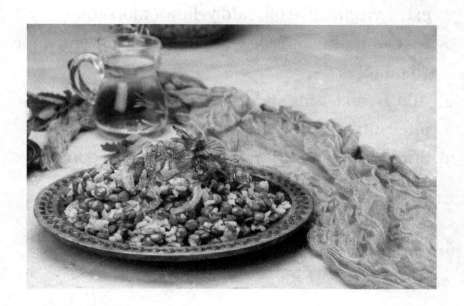

Ingredients

- 1/4 cup extra-virgin olive oil
- 1 large yellow onion, finely chopped
- 2 tsp. salt
- 2 cups green or brown lentils, picked over and rinsed
- 6 cups water
- 1 cup long-grain rice or brown rice

- 1 TB. Cumin

Directions

1. In a large, 3-quart pot over medium-low heat, heat extra-virgin olive oil. Add yellow onion and 1 teaspoon salt, and cook, stirring intermittently, for 10 minutes.
2. Add green lentils and water, and cook, stirring intermittently, for 20 minutes.
3. Stir in long-grain rice, remaining 1 teaspoon salt, and cumin. Cover and cook, stirring intermittently, for 40 minutes.
4. Serve warm or at room temperature with tzatziki sauce or a Mediterranean salad.

Gorgonzola And Chicken Pasta

Servings: 8 | Cooking: 40 min

Ingredients

- 12 oz pastas, cooked and drained
- ¼ cup snipped fresh Italian parsley
- 2/3 cup Parmesan cheese
- 1 cup crumbled Gorgonzola cheese
- 2 cups whipping cream
- 8 oz stemmed fresh cremini or shiitake mushrooms
- 3 tbsp olive oil
- ½ tsp ground pepper
- ½ tsp salt
- 1 ½ lbs. skinless chicken breast, cut into ½-inch slices

Directions

1. Season chicken breasts with ¼ tsp pepper and ¼ tsp salt.
2. On medium high fire, place a nonstick pan with 1 tbsp oil and stir fry half of the chicken until cooked and lightly browned, around 5 minutes per side.

Transfer chicken to a clean dish and repeat procedure to remaining batch of uncooked chicken.

3. In same pan, add a tablespoon of oil and stir fry mushroom until liquid is evaporated and mushrooms are soft, around eight minutes. Stir occasionally.

4. Add chicken back to the mushrooms along with cream and simmer for three minutes. Then add the remaining pepper and salt, parmesan cheese and ½ cup of Gorgonzola cheese. Cook until mixture is uniform. Turn off fire.

5. Add pasta into the mixture, tossing to combine. Transfer to serving dish and garnish with remaining Gorgonzola cheese and serve.

Nutrition: Calories: 358; Carbs: 23.1g; Protein: 27.7g; Fat: 17.1g

Pasta Shells Stuffed With Feta

Servings: 10 | Cooking: 40 min

Ingredients

- Cooking spray
- 20 jumbo pasta shells, cooked and drained
- 2 garlic cloves, minced
- 5 oz frozen chopped spinach, thawed, drained and squeezed dry
- 1 9oz package frozen artichoke hearts, thawed and chopped
- ¼ tsp freshly ground black pepper
- ½ cup fat free cream cheese softened
- 1 cup crumbled feta cheese
- 1 cup shredded provolone cheese, divided
- 1 8oz can no salt added tomato sauce
- 1 28oz can fire roasted crushed tomatoes with added puree
- ¼ cup chopped pepperoncini peppers
- 1 tsp dried oregano

Directions

1. On medium fire, place a medium fry pan and for 12 minutes cook tomato sauce, crushed tomatoes, peppers and oregano. Put aside.
2. In a medium bowl, mix garlic, spinach, artichoke, black pepper, cream cheese, feta cheese and ½ cup provolone. Evenly stuff these to the cooked pasta shells.
3. Grease a rectangular glass dish and arrange all the pasta shells within. Cover with tomato mixture and top with provolone.
4. Bake for 25 minutes in a preheated 375oF oven.

Nutrition: Calories: 284; Carbs: 38.5g; Protein: 15.9g; Fat: 8.3g

Kefta Styled Beef Patties With Cucumber Salad

Servings: 4 | Cooking: 10 min

Ingredients

- 2 pcs of 6-inch pita, quartered
- ½ tsp freshly ground black pepper
- 1 tbsp fresh lemon juice
- ½ cup plain Greek yogurt; fat free
- 2 cups thinly sliced English cucumber
- ½ tsp ground cinnamon
- ½ tsp salt
- 1 tsp ground cumin
- 2 tsp ground coriander
- 1 tbsp peeled and chopped ginger
- ¼ cup cilantro, fresh
- ¼ cup plus 2 tbsp fresh parsley, chopped and divided
- 1 lb. ground sirloin

Directions

1. On medium high fire, preheat a grill pan coated with cooking spray.
2. In a medium bowl, mix together cinnamon, salt, cumin, coriander, ginger, cilantro, parsley and beef. Then divide the mixture equally into four parts and shaping each portion into a patty ½ inch thick.
3. Then place patties on pan cooking each side for three minutes or until desired doneness is achieved.
4. In a separate bowl, toss together vinegar and cucumber.
5. In a small bowl, whisk together pepper, juice, 2 tbsp parsley and yogurt.
6. Serve each patty on a plate with ½ cup cucumber mixture and 2 tbsp of the yogurt sauce.

Nutrition: Calories per serving: 313; Carbs: 11.7g; Protein: 33.9g; Fat: 14.1g

Italian Mac & Cheese

Servings: 4 | Cooking: 6 min

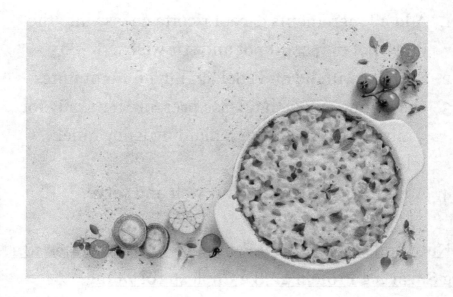

Ingredients

- 1 lb whole grain pasta
- 2 tsp Italian seasoning
- 1 1/2 tsp garlic powder
- 1 1/2 tsp onion powder
- 1 cup sour cream
- 4 cups of water
- 4 oz parmesan cheese, shredded
- 12 oz ricotta cheese

- Pepper
- Salt

Directions

1. Add all ingredients except ricotta cheese into the inner pot of instant pot and stir well.
2. Seal pot with lid and cook on high for 6 minutes.
3. Once done, allow to release pressure naturally for 5 minutes then release remaining using quick release. Remove lid.
4. Add ricotta cheese and stir well and serve.

Nutrition: Calories 388 Fat 25.8 g Carbohydrates 18.1 g Sugar 4 g Protein 22.8 g Cholesterol 74 mg

Saffron Green Bean-quinoa Soup

Servings: 6 | Cooking: 20 min

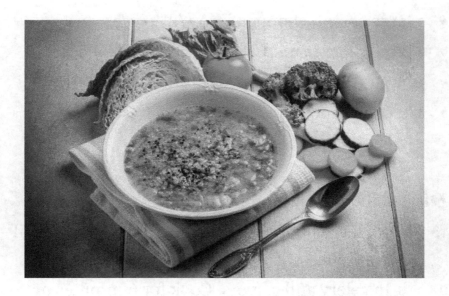

Ingredients

- 2 tablespoons extra virgin olive oil
- 1 large leek, white and light green parts only, halved, washed, and sliced
- 2 cloves garlic, minced
- 8 ounces fresh green beans, trimmed and chopped into 1" pieces
- 2 large pinches saffron, or one capsule
- 15 ounces chickpeas and liquid (do not rinse!)

- 1 large tomato, seeded and chopped into 1" pieces
- salt and freshly ground pepper, to taste
- freshly chopped basil, for serving
- 1 large carrot, chopped into 1/2" pieces
- 1 large celery stalk, chopped into 1/2" pieces
- 1 large zucchini, chopped into 1/2" pieces
- 1/2 cup quinoa, rinsed
- 4-5 cups vegetable stock

Directions

1. Place a large pot on medium fire and heat olive oil for 2 minutes.
2. Stir in celery and carrots. Cook for 6 minutes or until soft.
3. Mix in garlic and leek. Sauté for 3 minutes.
4. Add the zucchini and green beans, and sauté 1 minute more.
5. Pour in broth and saffron. Bring to a boil. Stir in chickpeas and quinoa. Cook until quinoa is soft, around 11 minutes while covered.
6. Stir in the diced tomato and salt and pepper, to taste, and remove from heat.

7. Serve the soup with the freshly chopped basil and enjoy!

Nutrition: Calories per serving: 196; Protein: 7.9g; Carbs: 26.6g; Fat: 7.5g

Black Bean Hummus

Servings: 8 | Cooking: 0 min

Ingredients

- 10 Greek olives
- ¼ tsp paprika
- ¼ tsp cayenne pepper
- ½ tsp salt
- ¾ tsp ground cumin
- 1 ½ tbsp tahini
- 2 tbsp lemon juice
- 1 15-oz can black beans, drain and reserve liquid
- 1 clove garlic

Directions

1. In food processor, mince garlic.
1. Add cayenne pepper, salt, cumin, tahini, lemon juice, 2 tbsp reserved black beans liquid, and black beans.
2. Process until smooth and creamy. Scrape the side of processor as needed and continue pureeing.
3. To serve, garnish with Greek olives and paprika.
4. Best eaten as a dip for pita bread or chips.

Nutrition: Calories per serving: 205; Protein: 12.1g; Carbs: 34.4g; Fat: 2.9g

Chapter 7: Dessert Recipes

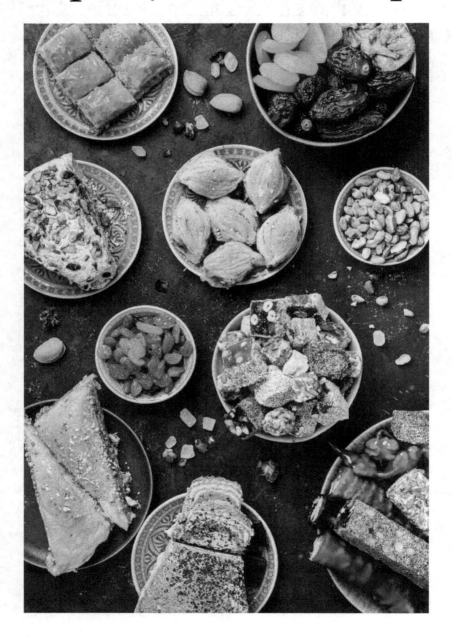

Lemon Cream

Servings: 6 | Cooking: 10 min

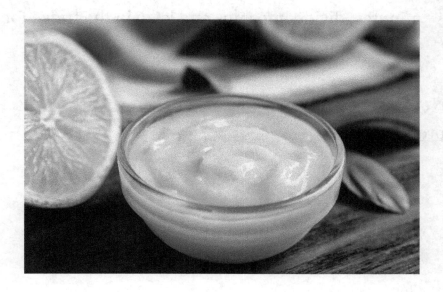

Ingredients

- 2 eggs, whisked
- 1 and ¼ cup stevia
- 10 tablespoons avocado oil
- 1 cup heavy cream
- Juice of 2 lemons
- Zest of 2 lemons, grated

Directions

1. In a pan, combine the cream with the lemon juice and the other ingredients, whisk well, cook for 10 minutes, divide into cups and keep in the fridge for 1 hour before serving.

Nutrition: calories 200; fat 8.5; fiber 4.5; carbs 8.6; protein 4.5

Sweet Tropical Medley Smoothie

Servings: 4 | Cooking: 5 min

Ingredients

- 1 banana, peeled
- 1 sliced mango
- 1 cup fresh pineapple
- ½ cup coconut water

Directions

2. Place all Ingredients in a blender.
3. Blend until smooth.
4. Pour in a glass container and allow to chill in the fridge for at least 30 minutes.

Nutrition: Calories per serving:73 ; Carbs: 18.6g; Protein: 0.8g; Fat: 0.5g.

Mediterranean Fruit Tart

Servings: 1/8 Of Tart | Cooking: 15 min

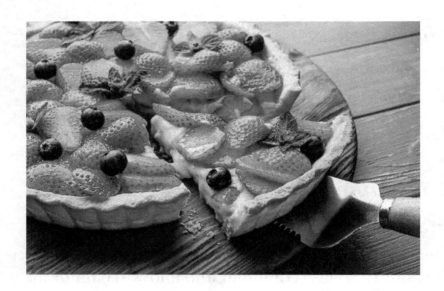

Ingredients

- 21/4 cups all-purpose flour
- 1/2 tsp. salt
- 2 TB. sugar
- 1 cup cold butter
- 1/2 cup shortening
- 5 TB. ice water
- 2 cups Ashta Custard (recipe earlier in this chapter)
- 10 strawberries, sliced

- 2 kiwi, peeled and sliced
- 1 cup blueberries
- 1 cup peach or apricot jam
- 3 TB. Water

Directions

1. In a food processor fitted with a chopping blade, pulse 2 cups all-purpose flour, salt, and sugar 5 times.
2. Add butter and shortening, and blend for 1 minute or until mixture is crumbly. Transfer mixture to a medium bowl.
3. Add ice water to batter, and mix just until combined.
4. Place dough on a piece of plastic wrap, form into a flat disc, and refrigerate for 20 minutes.
5. Preheat the oven to 450°F.
6. Dust your workspace with flour, and using a rolling pin, roll out dough to 1/8 inch thickness. Place rolled-out dough into a 9-inch tart pan, press to mold into pan, and cut off excess dough. Bake for 13 minutes.
7. Let tart cool for 10 minutes.

8. Place tart shell on a serving dish, and fill with Ashta Custard. Arrange strawberry slices, kiwi slices, and blueberries on top of tart.
9. In a small saucepan over medium heat, heat peach jam and water, stirring, for 2 minutes.
10.   Using a pastry brush, brush top of fruit and tart with warmed jam.
11. Serve chilled and store in the refrigerator.

Green Tea And Vanilla Cream

Servings: 4 | Cooking: 0 min

Ingredients

- 14 ounces almond milk, hot
- 2 tablespoons green tea powder
- 14 ounces heavy cream
- 3 tablespoons stevia
- 1 teaspoon vanilla extract
- 1 teaspoon gelatin powder

Directions

1. In a bowl, combine the almond milk with the green tea powder and the rest of the ingredients, whisk well, cool down, divide into cups and keep in the fridge for 2 hours before serving.

Nutrition: calories 120; fat 3; fiber 3; carbs 7; protein 4

Semolina Pie

Servings: 6 | Cooking: 1 Hour

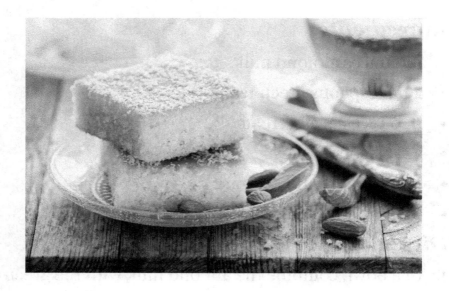

Ingredients

- ½ cup milk
- 3 tablespoons semolina
- ½ cup butter, softened
- 8 Phyllo sheets
- 2 eggs, beaten
- 3 tablespoons Erythritol
- 1 teaspoon lemon rind
- 1 tablespoon lemon juice

- 1 teaspoon vanilla extract
- 2tablespoons liquid honey
- 1 teaspoon ground cinnamon
- ¼ cup of water

Directions

1. Melt ½ part of all butter.
2. Then brush the casserole glass mold with the butter and place 1 Phyllo sheet inside.
3. Brush the Phyllo sheet with butter and cover it with second Phyllo sheet.
4. Make the dessert filling: heat up milk, and add semolina.
5. Stir it carefully.
6. After this, add remaining softened butter, Erythritol, and vanilla extract.
7. Bring the mixture to boil and simmer it for 2 minutes.
8. Remove it from the heat and cool to the room temperature.
9. Then add beaten eggs and mix up well.
10. Pour the semolina mixture in the mold over the Phyllo sheets, flatten it if needed.

11. Then cover the semolina mixture with remaining Phyllo sheets and brush with remaining melted butter.
12. Cut the dessert on the bars.
13. Bake galaktoboureko for 1 hour at 365F.
14. Then make the syrup: bring to boil lemon juice, honey, and water and remove the liquid from the heat.
15. Pour the syrup over the hot dessert and let it chill well.

Nutrition: calories 304; fat 18; fiber 1.1; carbs 39.4; protein 6.1

Vanilla Apple Compote

Servings: 6 | Cooking: 15 min

Ingredients

- 3 cups apples, cored and cubed
- 1 tsp vanilla
- 3/4 cup coconut sugar
- 1 cup of water
- 2 tbsp fresh lime juice

Directions

1. Add all ingredients into the inner pot of instant pot and stir well.
2. Seal pot with lid and cook on high for 15 minutes.
3. Once done, allow to release pressure naturally for 10 minutes then release remaining using quick release. Remove lid.
4. Stir and serve.

Nutrition: Calories 76 Fat 0.2 g Carbohydrates 19.1 g Sugar 11.9 g Protein 0.5 g Cholesterol 0 mg

Cold Lemon Squares

Servings: 4 | Cooking: 0 min

Ingredients

- 1 cup avocado oil+ a drizzle
- 2 bananas, peeled and chopped
- 1 tablespoon honey
- ¼ cup lemon juice
- A pinch of lemon zest, grated

Directions

1. In your food processor, mix the bananas with the rest of the ingredients, pulse well and spread on the bottom of a pan greased with a drizzle of oil.
2. Introduce in the fridge for 30 minutes, slice into squares and serve.

Nutrition: calories 136; fat 11.2; fiber 0.2; carbs 7; protein 1.1

Minty Coconut Cream

Servings: 2 | Cooking: 0 min

Ingredients

- 1 banana, peeled
- 2 cups coconut flesh, shredded
- 3 tablespoons mint, chopped
- 1 and ½ cups coconut water
- 2 tablespoons stevia
- ½ avocado, pitted and peeled

Directions

1. In a blender, combine the coconut with the banana and the rest of the ingredients, pulse well, divide into cups and serve cold.

Nutrition: calories 193; fat 5.4; fiber 3.4; carbs 7.6; protein 3

Cherry Cream

Servings: 4 | Cooking: 0 min

Ingredients

- 2 cups cherries, pitted and chopped
- 1 cup almond milk
- ½ cup whipping cream
- 3 eggs, whisked
- 1/3 cup stevia
- 1 teaspoon lemon juice
- ½ teaspoon vanilla extract

Directions

1. In your food processor, combine the cherries with the milk and the rest of the ingredients, pulse well, divide into cups and keep in the fridge for 2 hours before serving.

Nutrition: calories 200; fat 4.5; fiber 3.3; carbs 5.6; protein 3.4

Warm Peach Compote

Servings: 4 | Cooking: 1 Minute

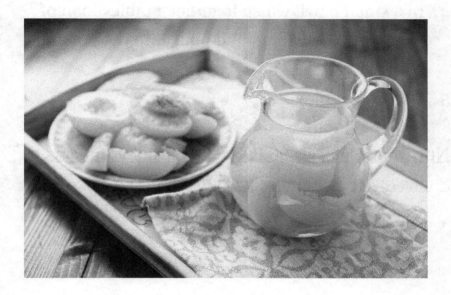

Ingredients

- 4 peaches, peeled and chopped
- 1 tbsp water
- 1/2 tbsp cornstarch
- 1 tsp vanilla

Directions

1. Add water, vanilla, and peaches into the instant pot.

2. Seal pot with lid and cook on high for 1 minute.
3. Once done, allow to release pressure naturally. Remove lid.
4. In a small bowl, whisk together 1 tablespoon of water and cornstarch and pour into the pot and stir well.
5. Serve and enjoy.

Nutrition: Calories 66 Fat 0.4 g Carbohydrates 15 g Sugar 14.1 g Protein 1.4 g Cholesterol 0 mg

Honey Walnut Bars

Servings: 8 | Cooking: 30 min

Ingredients

- 5 oz puff pastry
- ½ cup of water
- 3 tablespoons of liquid honey
- 1 teaspoon Erythritol
- 1/3 cup butter, softened
- ½ cup walnuts, chopped
- 1 teaspoon olive oil

Directions

1. Roll up the puff pastry and cut it on 6 sheets.
2. Then brush the tray with olive oil and arrange the first puff pastry sheet inside.
3. Grease it with butter gently and sprinkle with walnuts.
4. Repeat the same steps with 4 puff pastry sheets.
5. Then sprinkle the last layer with walnuts and Erythritol and cove with the sixth puff pastry sheet.
6. Cut the baklava on the servings.
7. Bake the baklava for 30 minutes.

8. Meanwhile, bring to boil liquid honey and water.
9. When the baklava is cooked, remove it from the oven.
10.   Pour hot honey liquid over baklava and let it cool till the room temperature.

Nutrition: calories 243; fat 19.6; fiber 0.8; carbs 15.9; protein 3.3

9 781803 257174